DENGUE FEVER

Strategies for Preventing Dengue and Bite Transmission via Mosquitoes

CARL JUAN

Table of Contents

Introductory

The dengue virus, which causes the disease, is spread to people mostly through the bites of infected female mosquitoes, especially the Aedes aegypti mosquito. Especially in tropical and subtropical areas, dengue fever poses a serious threat to public health.

• Dengue can cause mild to severe symptoms, the most common of which are high fever, severe headache, joint and muscular discomfort, rash, and a propensity to bleed. Dengue can cause severe bleeding, low blood pressure, and organ failure in some people, resulting in dengue hemorrhagic fever (DHF) or dengue shock syndrome (DSS).

• Since dengue cannot be cured with an antiviral drug, treatment concentrates on relieving symptoms and preventing complications. In high-risk locations, dengue can be avoided by eliminating breeding grounds for mosquitoes, applying insect repellent, and donning protective clothes.

• Public health programs to educate the public on dengue prevention and early symptom recognition are common components of efforts to limit the disease's distribution. In recent years, dengue vaccinations have been developed as an additional line of defense against the disease, albeit their availability and efficacy may vary by region.

CHAPTER ONE
Origins of Dengue Fever

Mosquitoes became the vector for the Dengue virus, which is thought to have started in primates and then spread to humans. The following is a synopsis of dengue's past:

• Dengue-like symptoms have been recorded in many places of the world dating back millennia. Dengue fever-like epidemics first appeared in Asia, the Caribbean, and Africa about 1779–1780. However, the dengue virus that causes the disease was not discovered until the twentieth century.

• The dengue virus was originally identified and isolated in the laboratory in 1943. Four different serotypes were identified and given the designations DEN-1, DEN-2, DEN-3, and DEN-4. Various virus subtypes can be traced back to these serotypes.

• Urbanization, population growth, and greater international travel all played a role in the global spread of dengue fever in the twentieth century. The principal vector for dengue, the Aedes aegypti mosquito, has expanded its range and become more common in many areas.

• Dengue hemorrhagic fever was originally identified in the 1950s in the Philippines and Thailand. The bleeding and low platelet count characteristic of DHF make it a potentially lethal variant of dengue.

• Many tropical and subtropical areas have been hit by dengue epidemics and outbreaks during the 20th and 21st centuries. In places with inadequate medical facilities, these epidemics can have catastrophic consequences.

• Over the years, scientists and health officials have labored to learn more about the dengue virus, its transmission, and the possibility of creating a vaccine against it. Public health initiatives and mosquito control operations have been launched in an effort to slow the virus's spread.

• Efforts to create a dengue vaccine have been ongoing for several decades. There have been multiple attempts to create and test a dengue vaccine, with variable degrees of success and availability in different parts of the world.

- Despite ongoing attempts to contain and prevent the disease, dengue fever continues to be a major global health problem in many regions. The continued spread and comeback of dengue in some locations can also be attributed to climate change and worldwide travel.

Dengue's long and widespread history is a product of the intricate relationship between viruses, ecosystems, and humans. Mosquito abatement, public awareness campaigns, and vaccination initiatives are the main tools in the fight against dengue.

The Spread of Dengue Virus

The dengue virus is a member of the Flaviviridae family of viruses and replicates only on a single strand of RNA. Female Aedes aegypti mosquitoes, which are responsible for most human infections, are the vectors for this virus. Here's a rundown of the ins and outs of the dengue virus's spread:

1. The dengue virus is a family of four related but distinct serotypes: DEN-1, DEN-2, DEN-3, and DEN-4. Getting infected with one serotype often results in lifetime immunity against that serotype, but not the others. Dengue hemorrhagic fever (DHF) and dengue shock syndrome (DSS) are both serious complications that can result from several infections with different serotypes.

2. The Aedes aegypti mosquito is the major carrier of the dengue virus. Another mosquito species, Aedes albopictus, can also spread the virus, albeit at a lower rate of success. These mosquitoes are commonly found in urban and semi-urban environments, and they feed during the day.

3. Dengue is spread when an infected individual is bitten by an

Aedes mosquito, which then bites someone else. Once infected, the mosquito can spread the disease to whoever it bites next. This pattern persists as long as there are mosquitoes carrying the disease.

4.Human-to-Mosquito

Transmission: When a person is infected with dengue, the virus can be present in their blood for a relatively short duration. During this viremic stage, the virus is present in the bloodstream and can be transmitted to a mosquito via a bite.

5. Infected mosquitoes can spread disease to humans by feeding on them after the virus has incubated in the insect for some time. The next step is to inject the virus directly into a person's veins.

6. In areas where Aedes mosquitoes are common and thrive, there is an increased risk of dengue transmission. Increased risk of dengue transmission may result from urbanization, high population density, and poor sanitation.

7. While mosquitoes are the most common way for dengue to spread, human-to-human transmission has been documented. This can occur by blood transfusion, organ transplantation, or from mother to kid during childbirth or breastfeeding.

8. Clinical Manifestations: After infection, dengue can present with symptoms ranging from mild flu-like symptoms to severe, potentially life-threatening diseases including dengue hemorrhagic fever (DHF) and dengue shock syndrome (DSS). The serotype of the virus and the host's immune system both play a role in determining the severity of the sickness.

Reducing mosquito breeding grounds, using insect repellents, and donning protective garments are the mainstays of dengue prevention. Dengue vaccinations have been produced in recent years to aid in protection against the virus, albeit their availability and efficacy may vary by region. Community education on dengue prevention and control is a focus of public health initiatives.

CHAPTER TWO
Dengue Symptoms in the Clinic

The severity of clinical symptoms associated with dengue fever might vary greatly. The severity of dengue fever can vary from person to person based on a number of factors, including the serotype of the dengue virus and the person's immune system. There are commonly three types of dengue clinical manifestations:

1. DF, or Dengue Fever

• High-grade fever: an acute onset of high-grade fever, typically up to 104°F (40°C).

Extreme pain in the head, most noticeably in the temples or the back of the head.

The discomfort felt in the muscles and joints is what gives dengue its alternative name, "breakbone fever."

• Soreness or pain in the area around or behind the eyes.

On the third or fifth day of illness, a rash may show up. It manifests as a rash of red patches (maculopapular) that may appear anywhere on the body.

Some people may have light bleeding, such a nosebleed or bleeding gums.

2. Symptoms of Dengue Fever

• Dengue fever can develop into Dengue Hemorrhagic Fever (DHF) in rare situations.

Dengue fever symptoms may include, but are not limited to, the following:

• Extreme discomfort in the gut

Recurrent vomiting

• Blood in the stool or vomit

Blood from the gums or nose

Petechiae (pink or red bumps) o Acne

3. Shock from a case of dengue fever:

The most severe form of dengue is known as Dengue Shock Syndrome, and it causes a dramatic drop in blood pressure, leading to shock.

All the symptoms of DHF apply to DSS as well as:

• A racing, feeble heartbeat

Cold, wet skin

An uneasy feeling

• Psychological change

If shock is not treated quickly, it can cause organ failure and death.

Not everyone who contracts the dengue virus will end up with the more severe forms of the illness (dengue fever or dengue shock syndrome). Most cases of dengue are rather mild and respond well to supportive therapy, including fluid replacement and pain medication. Severe instances, especially those with indications of DHF or DSS, require rapid medical attention and hospitalization.

A increased risk of severe dengue is seen in those who have already been infected with one serotype of the dengue virus but who then contract a second serotype. Therefore, in regions where dengue is endemic, it is vital to offer appropriate medical care and prevent serious sequelae by diagnosing and monitoring symptoms early.

Environmental, biological, and human variables all play a role in maintaining Dengue's cycle of transmission. The transmission of the dengue virus can be controlled and prevented if more people have a thorough understanding of these elements. **Some of the most**

important variables in dengue transmission are as follows:

• The Aedes aegypti mosquito, dengue's principal vector, plays a pivotal role in the disease's spread. The mosquito's susceptibility to infection and subsequent transmission to humans is crucial.

• Dengue transmission is highly sensitive to the population density of Aedes mosquitoes. High mosquito numbers increase the danger of virus transmission.

• Temperature and precipitation are two examples of climate and weather elements that might affect mosquito breeding, growth, and activity. Mosquitoes thrive in warm, damp conditions, which can increase the risk of transmission.

• Rapid urbanization and population increase can lead to squalor and stagnant water, ideal conditions for mosquito breeding. Dengue can also spread as a result of people traveling inside and between cities.

• Mosquito breeding grounds can be created by human actions such as inadequate sanitation, incorrect water storage, and poor waste disposal procedures. The danger of mosquito bites increases when people spend time outside without taking precautions (such as using insect repellent or wearing long sleeves and pants).

• Migration and travel can expose sick people or mosquitoes to new areas, allowing the virus to spread further. People with the virus can spread it to other locations with vulnerable people and appropriate vectors.

• Access to health care and standard of living are two examples of socioeconomic factors that may influence the severity of dengue outbreaks. Delays in diagnosing and treating severe dengue due to inadequate access to medical care may increase the risk of complications.

- Dengue infection risk factors include both current immunological state and previous infection history. While immunity to a single viral serotype may result from a previous infection, this protection does not extend to other virus serotypes. The severity of dengue fever can worsen if it is re-infected multiple times with various serotypes.

- **Vector Control Measures:** The success of vector control measures, such as mosquito eradication programs, usage of pesticides, and public health campaigns, can dramatically impact dengue transmission. Reducing mosquito populations and stopping their breeding is an important strategy for control.

• Dengue transmission can be affected by vaccination rates and vaccine accessibility. Dengue vaccinations have the potential to improve public health by reducing the number of infected people who can spread the virus outside the vaccinated population.

Public health initiatives, community engagement, environmental management, and improvements to healthcare facilities are often necessary to control and prevent dengue transmission. The impact of dengue in areas where it is endemic can be lessened by the use of coordinated efforts.

CHAPTER THREE
Laboratory and Medical Exams for Diagnosis

Clinical observation and laboratory tests are also necessary for a dengue diagnosis. Confirming a dengue infection, distinguishing it from other diseases with similar symptoms, and gauging the severity of the condition all depend on a proper diagnosis. The most reliable laboratory tests and diagnostic procedures for dengue are as follows:

• First, a doctor will conduct a clinical examination, which will involve looking at the patient's symptoms and past health records. High fever, headache, joint and muscle pain, a rash, and a propensity to bleed are all taken into account during the preliminary diagnosis of dengue.

• In the early stages of dengue infection, a fast diagnostic test is commonly performed using the NS1 (non-structural protein 1) antigen test. The NS1 protein, which is made by the dengue virus and can be found in the bloodstream within a few days of infection, is what this test looks for.

• The presence of dengue-specific antibodies in the blood can be determined by performing a serological test for IgM and IgG antibodies. In most cases, IgM antibodies can be detected a few days after the onset of symptoms and continue to be present for weeks. IgG antibodies are the result of a delayed immune response and may be detected for a longer time after a dengue infection has occurred.

• Direct detection of dengue virus DNA in a patient's blood can be achieved by the use of a molecular diagnostic test called reverse transcription polymerase chain reaction (RT-PCR). The viral RNA can be detected in its earliest stages because to the test's excellent sensitivity and specificity.

• **Hematological Tests:** Platelet count and hematocrit levels can be assessed with a complete blood count (CBC) and other blood tests to help determine the severity of dengue. Platelet count decreases and hematocrit rises as a result of severe dengue.

• **Isolation of the Virus:** The dengue virus can sometimes be extracted from a patient's blood or serum in a viral isolation lab. Although it is not frequently employed, virus isolation can give conclusive proof of dengue infection.

- Dengue can sometimes be diagnosed by a doctor using only clinical criteria and observation in areas where access to laboratory testing is limited. They keep an eye out for more serious dengue symptoms include a persistent vomiting, stomach pain, and blood.

Dengue should be diagnosed by a medical practitioner, and laboratory results should be interpreted in light of the patient's clinical presentation. Extreme forms of dengue (Dengue Hemorrhagic Fever and Dengue

Shock Syndrome) require prompt medical attention and an accurate diagnosis in order to be managed properly. Guidelines for the diagnosis and treatment of dengue fever are frequently issued by public health authorities in dengue-endemic regions.

Reducing the Spread of Dengue

Multiple approaches are needed to prevent and control dengue fever, all of which focus on lowering the spread of the virus. It is common for healthcare organizations, local governments, and communities to work together on these initiatives. The following are important measures for limiting the spread of dengue:

1. Directing a Vector:

• Dengue prevention efforts center around o Mosquito Control, the suppression of mosquito populations. Insecticide spraying, larviciding (the treatment of water containers where Aedes mosquitoes reproduce), and biological control approaches are all part of this strategy.

Communities need to work together to detect and eliminate containers, tires, and other standing water that could serve as mosquito breeding grounds.

2. Safeguarding Oneself:

• Using Mosquito Nets: Bed nets can be treated with pesticides to protect folks from mosquito bites while sleeping.

You can lessen your vulnerability to mosquito bites by taking preventative measures, such as donning long sleeves and pants and applying insect repellent.

• Fitting screens to entrances and windows will prevent mosquitoes from entering buildings.

3. Dengue prevention and the need of removing mosquito breeding areas can be highlighted in public education efforts.

Encourage local communities to organize cleanups and implement safety protocols.

4. Diagnosis and Treatment at an Early Stage:

• Medical personnel should be educated on how to spot dengue fever and make an accurate diagnosis.

Dengue cases can be treated more effectively if caught early, lowering the potential for serious complications.

5. Keeping an Eye on Things:

Understanding the local epidemiology of dengue requires constant monitoring of both dengue cases and mosquito populations.

• Monitoring can help identify epidemics and direct control actions.

6. Insect and Vector Control:

• To better manage mosquito populations, this strategy integrates environmental management, insecticide use, and community engagement.

7. Transit and Customs Procedures:

• Travel and migration can spread Dengue to new regions. The spread of the virus can be slowed or stopped by limiting the mobility of affected people and mosquitoes.

8. Dengue vaccinations have been developed and are suggested for those who are at a high risk of contracting the disease in certain geographic regions. The spread of dengue and the severity of its effects can be mitigated with vaccination.

9. Ecological Resource Administration:

• Mosquito breeding grounds can be reduced by using proper waste management and cleanliness precautions.

• Larvae buildup can be avoided by maintaining water storage containers and tanks on a regular basis.

10. Containing the Epidemic:

• In the event of a dengue outbreak, it is essential to take swift action, such as increasing efforts to eliminate vectors and provide medical care to those who have contracted the disease.

11. Discovery and Development:

• Dengue prevention, vaccine development, and vector control approaches must be studied continuously so that better strategies may be created.

The epidemiology of dengue fever varies from place to place, thus prevention and control measures need to be tailored to each individual area. Governments, healthcare providers, and communities must work together to effectively implement these strategies to lessen the impact of dengue and its sequelae.

'

CHAPTER FOUR
Controlling and Treating Dengue Fever

Dengue requires primarily supportive therapy to ease symptoms, track complications, and guarantee enough hydration. More intensive medical intervention is required in cases of severe dengue, which includes dengue hemorrhagic fever (DHF) and dengue shock syndrome (DSS).

1. Care for Moderate Dengue:

• Recovery from dengue requires rest, therefore sick people should get lots of it.

To avoid becoming dehydrated, it is essential to drink enough water throughout the day. Maintaining hydration through the consumption of oral rehydration solutions (ORS), water, and other clear fluids is recommended.

Fever and pain can be treated with over-the-counter medications such acetaminophen (paracetamol). If you're at danger of bleeding, you should avoid using non-steroidal anti-inflammatory medicines (NSAIDs) like ibuprofen.

2. Symptom Tracking:

• Even in mild cases of dengue, regular symptom monitoring is crucial. If your symptoms get worse, it's time to see a doctor.

3. Diagnostic Procedures:

• Individuals with dengue should seek medical assessment to confirm the diagnosis and determine the severity of the condition. The most effective treatment is achieved with a prompt diagnosis

4. Hospitalization is often required for patients with dengue hemorrhagic fever or dengue shock syndrome.

Blood pressure and shock can be avoided with the help of fluid replacement therapy. To restore fluid balance, intravenous (IV) fluids are given.

5. Transfusion of Blood:

• Transfusions of blood or platelets may be necessary in extreme circumstances to control excessive bleeding and a low platelet count.

6. Checking the Hematocrit Level:

• Hematocrit, the percentage of blood volume occupied by red blood cells, should be measured on a regular basis. When the hematocrit rises dramatically, it may be because plasma is leaking out and more fluid needs to be replaced.

7. Medical Emergency:

• Dengue shock syndrome patients who develop potentially fatal complications may require round-the-clock observation in an ICU.

8. Treatment of Pain and Other Symptoms:

• Medication is used for pain, nausea, and other symptoms as required.

9. Limiting the Spread of Germs:

• Secondary bacterial infections, which can worsen dengue cases, are avoided with preventative measures. Antibiotics and other forms of good hygiene may be required.

10. Keep an Eye Out for Problems:

• Improving patient outcomes requires prompt diagnosis and management of complications such life-threatening hemorrhage, organ failure, or shock.

11. Nutrition:

• Recuperation is aided by eating well. If at all feasible, patients should be urged to eat healthily.

Early management can reduce the progression to severe dengue in people with suspected or confirmed dengue, especially those who experience severe symptoms or warning indications. Because of the severity of its symptoms, dengue fever requires close medical supervision and treatment in areas where it is endemic. Healthcare providers can often find instructions for treating dengue fever online, written by public health agencies in impacted regions.

Precautions for One's Own Safety

The chance of contracting an illness like dengue, which is spread by mosquitoes, can be greatly reduced by taking precautions against being bitten. These precautions should not be ignored in dengue hotspots.

In order to avoid contracting dengue fever, you can take the following preventative measures:

1. Applying DEET (N,N-diethyl-m-toluamide) or another effective insect repellent on exposed skin is a good way to keep mosquitoes at bay. For optimal results, use as directed by the manufacturer.

2. At dusk and dawn, when mosquitoes are most active, it's best to cover up with long sleeves and pants.

Permethrin-treated garments offer an extra layer of defense.

3. You can reduce your risk of being bitten by mosquitoes by staying in places that have screens on the windows and doors or by turning on the air conditioner.

4. In order to prevent dengue fever while you sleep, it is recommended that you wear an insecticide-treated mosquito net.

5. Prevent Being Bit During Mosquito Peak:

• The dengue virus is spread mostly by Aedes mosquitoes, which are most active in the morning and late afternoon. Avoid going outside as much as possible during this time.

If you absolutely have to go outside, arm yourself with repellant and protective gear.

6. Get Rid of Mosquito Habitats

• Containers, flowerpots, and open water storage containers are all potential mosquito breeding locations, so it's important to monitor your environment on a regular basis.

To stop mosquitoes from breeding, you should get rid of standing water, cover containers, or use larvicides.

7.You can prevent mosquitoes from entering your home by installing screens on all of the entrances and windows.

8. Gutter cleaning and maintenance is important because blocked gutters can lead to mosquito breeding ponds. Maintaining clean and functional gutters will keep water from pooling.

9. Avoid keeping water in open containers for long periods of time. Keep any containers used to store water securely covered.

10. Since mosquitoes can lay their eggs in very small containers, such as pet water bowls, it's important to regularly clean and replace them.

Keep these containers clean and replenish the water in them frequently.

11. Community Engagement: Encourage your community to engage in clean-up drives and the elimination of breeding places. Preventing dengue through community actions has the potential to be very successful.

12. Get the word out about the need of personal protection measures and how to prevent dengue in yourself and your community.

When utilized regularly and in conjunction with community-wide initiatives to minimize mosquito breeding areas, personal protection techniques can be quite successful. Dengue prevention relies heavily on lowering mosquito populations and protecting people from mosquito bites, particularly in areas where the disease is a major public health issue.

Conclusion

Infected Aedes mosquitoes, especially Aedes aegypti, are the primary vectors for spreading the dengue virus to humans. Dengue fever, a mild form of the disease, can progress to dengue hemorrhagic fever (DHF) and dengue shock syndrome (DSS), both potentially fatal conditions. Environmental, ecological, and human variables all play a role in dengue transmission, making it a challenging public health issue.

Vector control techniques, personal protection, community engagement, and early detection and diagnosis are all key components in the battle against dengue. Supportive care, such as fluid replacement and blood transfusions, are used to treat mild instances of dengue fever, whereas more intense medical interventions are used to treat severe cases.

The risk of infection can be greatly reduced with the use of personal protective measures such insect repellents, protective clothing, and the elimination of mosquito breeding areas. Dengue is a mosquito-borne disease, and attempts to prevent and manage it are continuous and necessitate cooperation between governments, healthcare authorities, communities, and individuals. The global effort to combat dengue fever relies heavily on public awareness, education, and research.

THE END